Copyright Page for "Remember Me"

Remember Me
Written by Wesley Wren

Copyright © 2024 by Wesley Wren
All rights reserved.

Published by 150th Publishing
Monee, Illinois, USA

No part of this book may be reproduced, distributed, or transmitted in any form or by any means, including photocopying, recording, or other electronic or mechanical methods, without the prior written permission of the author, except in the case of brief quotations embodied in critical reviews and certain other noncommercial uses permitted by copyright law.

For permission requests, write to the publisher at the address below:

150th Publishing
Monee IL

Showtimemusicgroup.com

This is a work of fiction. Names, characters, places, and incidents either are the product of the author's imagination or are used fictitiously. Any resemblance to actual persons, living or dead, events, or locales is entirely coincidental.

ISBN: 9798302775818

Printed in the United States of America

First Edition: 2024

Remember Me?

Wesley Wren

150th Publishing

For Leon "PaPa" Williams

Willow Grove Nursing Home

The first rays of sunlight streamed through the large, lace-curtained windows of Willow Grove Nursing Home, casting golden patterns across the polished linoleum floors. Outside, the world was waking up. Birds chirped in the oak trees lining the driveway, and a light breeze rustled the leaves, carrying the earthy smell of dew into the building. Inside, the nursing home was already a hive of activity, even though most of the residents were still tucked away in their rooms.

Annie, a young caregiver in her mid-twenties with auburn hair tied back in a loose ponytail, was the first to arrive in the dining room that morning. She carried a tray laden with pitchers of orange juice, milk, and water. Her sneakers squeaked softly as she moved across the floor, arranging the pitchers on the sideboard near the coffee urn. The aroma of freshly brewed coffee was just beginning to fill the air, mingling with the faint smell of disinfectant that never quite disappeared.

"Another day, another adventure," Annie muttered under her breath, half-smiling as she glanced at the neatly arranged dining tables. Each was covered with a white tablecloth and set with cheerful, yellow plates and cups that contrasted the gray walls of the room.

She knew what lay ahead. Every day at Willow Grove was a mixture of heartwarming moments, small victories, and heartbreaks. Annie often thought of the residents as an extended family—each of them with their own quirks, struggles, and stories. This morning, as she adjusted a slightly askew centerpiece on one of the tables, she found herself thinking about them.

Sarah would likely be the first to arrive, shuffling in with her walker and her usual cheerful smile. Annie could already imagine her saying, "Good morning, sunshine," in her sing-song voice. Sarah was always cheerful in the mornings, though the same couldn't be said for later in the day when her Alzheimer's would sometimes confuse her or leave her agitated.

John would follow not long after. A retired postal worker with vascular dementia, he liked to sit by the window and sip his coffee while working on a crossword puzzle. Except, lately, his crosswords had become more of a guessing game. Still, he tackled them with determination, a look of concentration furrowing his brow.

And then there was Linda, the former artist with Lewy body dementia. Mornings were always unpredictable with Linda. Sometimes she'd burst into the room wide-eyed, insisting that birds or strange shapes had been floating outside her window. Other days, she'd be quieter, retreating into a world of her own.

Annie moved to the coffee urn, checking the level. The machine gurgled softly, promising a fresh batch soon. She glanced at her watch—6:45 a.m. Breakfast trays would be wheeled out in fifteen minutes. She liked this time of day, the calm before the storm.

"Good morning, Annie," a voice called from the doorway, interrupting her thoughts. It was Maria, the head nurse, her arms full of files and her face already wearing its usual expression of gentle efficiency. Maria had been working at Willow Grove for over a decade and seemed to know every resident's quirks, preferences, and history by heart.

"Morning, Maria," Annie replied, pouring herself a small cup of coffee. "Ready for another day?"

Maria chuckled softly. "I don't know if I'm ready, but it's here whether I like it or not. Let's just hope Edward doesn't decide to reorganize the kitchen again."

The two women laughed, though the memory of Edward's impromptu kitchen raid a few days ago was still fresh. Edward, a former bakery owner with frontotemporal dementia, often acted impulsively. That morning, he'd decided the spice rack needed a complete overhaul, mixing oregano with cinnamon and hiding the pepper shakers in the freezer.

"Speaking of Edward, is he still asleep?" Annie asked, leaning against the counter.

"For now," Maria said with a knowing smile. "But you know he's an early riser. He'll probably be up and about before breakfast is even served."

Annie nodded, taking a sip of her coffee. Her mind wandered to the other residents. Margaret, with her mixed dementia, often got lost on her way to the dining room and would need gentle guidance. Henry, the musician with Parkinson's disease dementia, would shuffle in later, his harmonica always close at hand. Emily, whose Huntington's disease left her movements unsteady, would need help with her utensils during breakfast. And Robert—poor Robert—was slipping away faster than anyone wanted to admit. Creutzfeldt-Jakob disease was cruel, stealing him from them bit by bit, even though he was still physically present.

She sighed, setting her coffee down. "It's hard sometimes, isn't it? Watching them fade."

Maria gave her a sympathetic look. "It is. But think of the moments we bring them—those small, bright spots in their day. That's why we're here, Annie."

Annie nodded, her resolve strengthened. She glanced at the clock again—7:00 a.m. It was time to get the show on the road.

By 7:15, the dining room was bustling with activity. Sarah was indeed the first to arrive, her walker scraping softly against the floor as she made her way to her favorite table near the window.

"Good morning, sunshine!" she called out, her voice filled with warmth.

"Good morning, Sarah," Annie replied, smiling. "How are you feeling today?"

"Like a spring chicken," Sarah said with a laugh, settling into her chair. Annie placed a glass of orange juice in front of her, and Sarah immediately began chatting about the weather, her words tumbling out like water over rocks.

John entered next, his cane tapping rhythmically as he moved to his usual spot. Annie handed him his crossword puzzle and a pencil, and he nodded his thanks, already deep in thought as he sipped his coffee.

A commotion at the door signaled Linda's arrival. She paused, looking around the room with a puzzled expression.

"Annie," she said, her voice low, "do you see them? The birds—they're everywhere!"

Annie walked over, placing a gentle hand on Linda's arm. "I don't see them, but maybe they flew out to the garden. Would you like to sit by the window and keep an eye out for them?"

Linda nodded hesitantly, allowing Annie to guide her to a seat near Sarah. As she sat down, her gaze softened, and she began talking about a painting she once made of a bluebird. Sarah, always eager for conversation, chimed in, and soon the two women were chatting like old friends.

By mid-morning, the dining room had emptied, and the residents were scattered throughout the home. Some attended a morning exercise class in the activity room, while others lingered in the garden or retreated to their rooms for some quiet time.

Annie took a moment to catch her breath, leaning against the counter in the nurses' station. The morning rush was over, but the day was just beginning. She thought about how each resident brought something unique to Willow Grove. Sarah's warmth, John's determination, Linda's artistic soul—they all contributed to the tapestry of life here.

She also thought about how their lives intertwined in subtle ways. Sarah's cheerfulness often lifted Linda's spirits. John's crossword puzzles sometimes sparked memories for Margaret. And even Edward's impulsive antics, though challenging, often brought unexpected laughter to the staff and residents.

Annie smiled to herself. Willow Grove wasn't just a nursing home—it was a community, a family. And even though some days were harder than others, she couldn't imagine being anywhere else.

As she walked back to the dining room to prepare for lunch, she thought about something Maria had said earlier: "Think of the moments we bring them." Annie vowed to make today full of moments—bright, meaningful, unforgettable moments.

Because here, at Willow Grove, even when memories faded, love and connection remained.

Chapter 1: Sarah

The sun had climbed higher in the sky, casting warm light across the soft beige walls of Willow Grove Nursing Home. Sarah shuffled into the activity room after breakfast, humming an old tune under her breath. Her walker squeaked with every step, a rhythm that matched her cheerful demeanor. She wore her usual pale blue cardigan, its edges lightly frayed, and a floral brooch pinned neatly to her collar.

"Good morning, sunshine!" she chirped to no one in particular, her voice carrying through the room.

Annie, standing by the activity board, smiled. Sarah's optimism was infectious, even if it came with the forgetfulness of her Alzheimer's. Every day was a new start for Sarah, sometimes for better, sometimes for worse. Today, it seemed, was one of her better days.

"Good morning, Sarah," Annie replied, walking over to help her settle into a chair. "You're looking bright-eyed and bushy-tailed this morning."

"Why wouldn't I be?" Sarah said with a chuckle, patting Annie's hand. "It's a beautiful day, and I've got so much to do."

Annie nodded, knowing well that "so much to do" often meant sorting through the same photo album multiple times or rearranging the knickknacks on her bedside table. Still, she didn't mind humoring Sarah. "What's first on your agenda today?"

"Well, I thought I might teach a little bit," Sarah said, her tone serious now. "The children will be waiting, you know."

Annie's chest tightened. Sarah often slipped back into her old role as a schoolteacher, forgetting that she had retired decades ago. "Oh, I'm sure they'd love that," Annie said gently. "What subject are you teaching today?"

"Reading, of course," Sarah replied, her eyes twinkling. "It's the most important skill, you know. You can't get anywhere in life without reading."

"Absolutely," Annie agreed. "Why don't we find you a book to look through? Maybe you can decide what to read to the class."

Sarah nodded enthusiastically as Annie fetched a worn hardcover from the bookshelf. It was a children's book with colorful illustrations, one Sarah had read dozens of times before. Sarah took the book in her hands, tracing her fingers over the cover.

"Oh, this one," she said, smiling. "This was always a favorite in my class."

She opened the book and began reading aloud, her voice steady and clear. As she read, other residents drifted into the room. Some paused to listen, while others moved to different corners to work on puzzles or crafts. Sarah didn't seem to notice the audience growing around her; she was completely absorbed in the story.

By mid-morning, Sarah had finished the book and was sitting quietly, gazing out the window. Annie approached her with a cup of tea, placing it on the table in front of her.

"Thank you, dear," Sarah said, her voice softer now. She seemed less sure of herself, as though the clarity of earlier had slipped away.

"Are you okay?" Annie asked, sitting down beside her.

Sarah nodded but didn't meet Annie's eyes. "I just... I feel like I've forgotten something important. Do you ever feel like that?"

Annie hesitated, unsure how to respond. "Sometimes," she said finally. "But usually, it's nothing too important. And if it is, it always comes back to me eventually."

Sarah looked at her, her brow furrowed. "Do you think they're angry with me? The children?"

"Angry? Why would they be angry?" Annie asked.

"For not showing up to class," Sarah said, her voice trembling. "I think... I think I was supposed to be there today."

Annie reached out, covering Sarah's hand with her own. "No one's angry, Sarah. I promise. And you've already done so much teaching today. You read that wonderful story, didn't you?"

Sarah seemed to relax at that, her shoulders loosening. "I suppose you're right. It was a good story, wasn't it?"

"It was," Annie said with a smile. "You're still a wonderful teacher, Sarah."

For a moment, Sarah seemed at peace. She sipped her tea, her gaze returning to the window. Annie stayed beside her, silently watching as a robin hopped along the garden path outside.

Later that day, Sarah wandered into the hallway, her walker clattering softly against the floor. She paused in front of a bulletin board filled with photos and announcements. One picture caught her eye—a group photo of the residents and staff from last summer's garden party. Sarah leaned in, squinting at the image.

"Is that... me?" she asked, her voice barely above a whisper.

Annie, passing by, stopped to look. "It is. That was from our garden party last year. Do you remember it?"

Sarah shook her head, her expression a mixture of curiosity and sadness. "I don't. But I look happy."

"You were," Annie said. "It was a beautiful day. You wore your pink hat, the one with the flowers, and you danced in the garden."

"I danced?" Sarah said, a flicker of joy in her eyes. "I used to love dancing."

"You still do," Annie said. "And you were wonderful that day. Everyone was watching you."

Sarah smiled faintly, her fingers brushing the edge of the photo. "I wish I could remember it."

Annie didn't know what to say. Moments like this were the hardest—when the gaps in Sarah's memory became too wide to bridge. But Annie also knew that the emotions of the moment—the joy, the connection—were more important than the details.

"Maybe we'll have another garden party soon," Annie said, her voice bright. "And you can dance again."

"I'd like that," Sarah said, her smile growing. "I'd like that very much."

As the day wore on, Sarah moved between activities, her energy dipping but her cheerfulness never completely fading. By dinner, she was seated with Linda and John at a table near the window. They chatted about little things—Linda's birds, John's crossword puzzle—while Sarah occasionally chimed in with a comment or a laugh.

Annie watched from across the room, feeling a swell of affection for Sarah. Despite the challenges of her Alzheimer's, Sarah had a way of bringing warmth to those around her. She didn't always remember the details, but she remembered how to make people feel loved and valued.

As the sun set and the residents began retreating to their rooms for the night, Annie helped Sarah back to hers. She tucked Sarah in, smoothing the blanket over her shoulders.

"Goodnight, Sarah," she said softly. "Sleep well."

"Goodnight, sunshine," Sarah replied, her eyes already closing.

Annie stood by the door for a moment, watching as Sarah's breathing slowed and she drifted off to sleep. The day had been a good one, Annie thought. Sarah might not remember it tomorrow, but that didn't matter. What mattered was that, for today, she had been happy.

And that was enough.

Chapter 2: John

John's day began the way it always did: with the soft shuffle of slippers across the floor and the rhythmic tap of his cane against the linoleum. At seventy-two, John prided himself on maintaining his independence as much as possible, even if vascular dementia had slowed him down considerably. This morning, like every other, he made his way to the dining room with purpose, though his mind wandered as he walked.

He reached the dining room a few minutes before breakfast was served. The aroma of coffee and toast greeted him, stirring a distant memory of mornings spent with his late wife, Martha. She'd always insisted on fresh coffee, and the smell of it would fill their little kitchen as she buttered toast and read the newspaper aloud.

John blinked, the memory slipping away almost as quickly as it had come. He settled into his usual seat by the window, nodding a polite hello to Sarah, who was already chatting animatedly with Annie about the birds outside. John's attention, however, was focused on the folded newspaper waiting for him on the table. Tucked neatly beside it was his daily crossword puzzle.

John's love of crosswords had been a lifelong habit, one he refused to give up even as dementia made the task more difficult. He unfolded the page and picked up his pencil, his fingers trembling slightly. The first clue stared back at him: "Four-letter word for a famous Egyptian queen."

"Easy," John muttered to himself. "Cleopatra."

He wrote the word in the blank squares, but by the time he finished, doubt crept in. Was Cleopatra the right answer? Or was it Nefertiti? The thought spun in his mind, scattering the focus he'd started with. Frustrated, he erased the letters, leaving a smudge behind.

"Need some help, John?" Annie asked as she approached with his coffee.

John shook his head. "No, no. I've got it. Just a little rusty, that's all."

Annie smiled knowingly but didn't press him. She set the coffee down and moved on, leaving John to wrestle with the puzzle. He worked through a few more clues, some successfully, others less so. "A two-letter word for agreement," he mumbled. "A-Y-E. Aye."

Satisfied with his answer, he moved on, though he still glanced out the window every so often, his thoughts drifting.

By mid-morning, John was in the activity room, still holding his crossword puzzle. Today's group activity was a light exercise class, but John had little interest in joining. Instead, he chose a seat by the far wall, where he could watch without participating.

As Annie led the group through gentle stretches, John continued to stare at his crossword. The clues were becoming harder, and the answers that once came to him effortlessly now danced just out of reach. He clenched his pencil tighter, willing his brain to cooperate.

"Having trouble, John?" a voice asked, startling him. He looked up to see Margaret, her kind face framed by a cascade of silver hair. She carried a book in her hands, but her gaze was fixed on his puzzle.

"Just a bit," John admitted. "Can't seem to get the hang of this one today."

Margaret nodded and pulled up a chair beside him. "Let me see. Maybe I can help."

John hesitated. He didn't like asking for help—it felt like admitting defeat—but Margaret's smile was gentle and unassuming. He handed her the crossword reluctantly

"Let's see," she said, scanning the clues. "Ah, here's one. 'Five-letter word for a flightless bird.' That's easy. It's 'ostrich.'"

John watched as she filled in the squares with steady hands. "I would've gotten that," he muttered.

"Of course you would have," Margaret said, handing the puzzle back. "Sometimes it just helps to have a fresh pair of eyes."

John grunted in acknowledgment, though he couldn't deny that her help had given him a small sense of relief.

Later in the afternoon, John found himself in the garden, his crossword abandoned for now. The crisp autumn air was invigorating, and he liked the quiet of the outdoor space. He walked slowly along the stone path, his cane clicking against the ground.

He paused by a wooden bench, lowering himself onto it with care. From here, he had a clear view of the bird feeder that hung from an old oak tree. A small sparrow darted in and out, pecking at the seeds.

"Used to be a mailman, you know," John said aloud, as if addressing the bird. "Walked this much and more every day. Rain, snow, didn't matter."

The sparrow didn't respond, of course, but talking to it made John feel a little less lonely. He leaned back on the bench, closing his eyes for a moment. The sound of the wind rustling through the leaves reminded him of the neighborhoods he used to walk through, the friendly faces he'd see along his route. He wondered if they remembered him.

By early evening, John was back in the dining room for dinner. The crossword puzzle lay forgotten on the table beside his plate of meatloaf and mashed potatoes. Across from him, Sarah was telling Linda about a story she had read to a class earlier in the day. John listened half-heartedly, more interested in his food.

After dinner, Annie approached him with a gentle smile. "Did you finish your puzzle, John?"

"Not quite," he admitted. "It's harder than it looks."

"Well, maybe we can take a look at it together tomorrow," Annie suggested. "Fresh eyes, right?"

John chuckled, the phrase reminding him of Margaret's earlier assistance. "Fresh eyes," he echoed. "Maybe you're onto something."

Annie took his tray and gave his shoulder a reassuring pat. "Goodnight, John."

"Goodnight, Annie," he said, his voice softer now. He stayed at the table a little longer, gazing out the window as the last traces of daylight faded into the horizon.

When John finally returned to his room, he placed the unfinished crossword puzzle on his bedside table. He didn't like leaving things undone, but tonight, he was too tired to care. As he lay back against the pillows, his thoughts drifted once again to Martha and their mornings together. He could almost hear her voice, clear and steady, reading the newspaper aloud.

"Four-letter word for an Egyptian queen," he murmured, his eyelids growing heavy. This time, the answer came to him easily.

"Cleopatra," he whispered, a faint smile on his lips as he drifted off to sleep.

Chapter 3: Linda

Linda awoke to a room awash in pale morning light, streaming through the slats of the blinds. She blinked, trying to focus her gaze on the ceiling above her. It took her a moment to remember where she was. Her room at Willow Grove Nursing Home was neat and simple, but sometimes it felt unfamiliar. Today was one of those days.

She sat up slowly, her body stiff from sleep, and swung her legs over the side of the bed. The faint sound of birds chirping outside her window caught her attention, and her lips curled into a small smile.

Birds. They were always there, keeping her company.

Linda shuffled to the window and peered out, her hands gripping the windowsill. There they were—little brown sparrows hopping along the garden path. But as she watched, her heart skipped. She could swear there was something else among the birds—a flicker of bright blue, darting in and out of view. A bluebird? No, it was too big for that. It looked almost like...

"A parrot," she whispered, her voice trembling. Her mind reeled as the vibrant image took root. Yes, she was sure of it now. A parrot, perched just beyond the garden, watching her with intelligent eyes.

She turned away from the window and reached for her robe. "I have to tell someone," she murmured.

By the time Linda arrived in the dining room, breakfast was in full swing. The clatter of dishes and the hum of conversation filled the air, but Linda's focus remained singular. She scanned the room until her eyes landed on Annie, who was pouring coffee at a nearby table.

"Annie," Linda called, her voice a mixture of urgency and excitement. "You'll never believe what I saw!"

Annie turned, her face lighting up. "Good morning, Linda. What did you see?"

"A parrot," Linda said, gripping Annie's arm. "Out in the garden. A beautiful, blue parrot."

Annie blinked, her smile faltering for only a moment before she recovered. "A parrot? That's unusual. Are you sure?"

"Of course, I'm sure," Linda insisted. "It was right there, watching me."

Annie nodded, her tone gentle. "Maybe it escaped from somewhere nearby. Would you like to sit by the window and keep an eye out for it?"

Linda hesitated. Part of her wanted to go back outside and find the bird herself, but the idea of sitting by the window and watching felt safer. "Yes, I'd like that."

Annie led her to a table near the window and poured her a cup of tea. "There you go. Let me know if you see it again."

Linda nodded, her eyes already scanning the garden. The sparrows were still there, pecking at the ground, but the parrot was gone. She sipped her tea, her hands trembling slightly. She couldn't shake the feeling that the bird had been real, that it had come to tell her something important.

After breakfast, Linda wandered into the activity room. The morning sunlight streamed through the large windows, casting warm patches of light across the floor. A few residents were already gathered, working on puzzles or chatting quietly. Linda chose a seat near the window, where she could keep watch for the parrot.

Annie appeared a few minutes later, carrying a tray of art supplies. "Linda, I thought you might like to paint today," she said, setting the tray down on the table.

Linda's eyes lit up. Painting was one of the few things that still brought her joy. Even on her worst days, when the fog in her mind felt impenetrable, the feel of a paintbrush in her hand was like a lifeline.

"I'd like that," she said, reaching for the brushes.

Annie laid out a sheet of paper and a palette of colors. "What will you paint today?" she asked.

"The parrot," Linda said without hesitation.

She dipped her brush into the blue paint and began to work. As the brush glided across the paper, the image in her mind grew sharper. The parrot's wings were outstretched, its feathers shimmering with hues of blue and green. Its eyes were piercing and wise, as though it held the secrets of the world.

Linda worked in silence, her focus unbroken. When she finally stepped back to admire her painting, a sense of pride swelled in her chest. She hadn't felt this way in a long time.

"That's beautiful," Annie said, leaning over to look. "You're so talented, Linda."

Linda smiled faintly, her gaze still on the painting. "Do you think it's real?" she asked, her voice barely above a whisper.

Annie hesitated, choosing her words carefully. "I think it's real to you, and that's what matters."

Linda nodded, though her mind still clung to the image of the parrot. She wondered where it had gone, and whether it would come back.

By mid-afternoon, Linda had taken her painting back to her room and propped it up on her nightstand. She lay on her bed, staring at it, the vibrant colors almost alive against the stark white background.

Her mind drifted, and memories surfaced—disjointed, fragmented. She remembered a different time, long before Willow Grove, when her world had been filled with color and life. She had been an artist, a painter whose work hung in galleries. People had admired her, sought her out for her vision and creativity. But that life felt distant now, like a dream she couldn't quite recall.

A knock on the door brought her back to the present. Annie peeked in, her smile warm. "Hi, Linda. How are you doing?"

Linda gestured to the painting. "Do you think I should show it to the others?"

"I think they'd love that," Annie said. "Why don't we bring it to the common room?"

Linda hesitated but nodded. With Annie's help, she carried the painting to the common room, where a small group of residents was gathered. Sarah was there, chatting with Margaret, and John was sitting quietly with his crossword.

"Look at what Linda painted," Annie announced, holding up the painting.

The residents murmured in admiration, their faces lighting up as they took in the vibrant colors. Sarah clapped her hands. "Oh, it's wonderful, Linda! So bright and lively."

John squinted at the painting, his brow furrowing. "A parrot, is it?"

"Yes," Linda said, her voice firm. "I saw it this morning. Out in the garden."

"Maybe it was just passing through," John said, his tone thoughtful. "Birds do that, you know. They come and go."

Linda nodded, though a part of her didn't believe the parrot had simply "passed through." She felt it had come for a reason, though she couldn't quite explain why.

As the day drew to a close, Linda sat by her window, the painting resting on her lap. The sun was setting, casting a warm golden light across the garden. The sparrows were still there, hopping along the path, but the parrot was nowhere to be seen.

Linda sighed, her fingers tracing the edge of the painting. Maybe John was right. Maybe the parrot had simply been passing through. Or maybe it had been a figment of her imagination, a trick played by her own mind.

But as the last rays of sunlight disappeared, Linda felt a strange sense of peace. Whether the parrot was real or not didn't matter. What mattered was the feeling it had left behind—the spark of creativity, the sense of wonder. For the first time in a long while, Linda felt like herself again.

"Goodnight," she whispered, as if speaking to the parrot. She set the painting on her nightstand and climbed into bed, her heart lighter than it had been in months.

And as she drifted off to sleep, she dreamed of wings and skies filled with color.

Chapter 4: Edward

Edward woke up before the sun, as he always did. He lay in his bed for a moment, staring at the ceiling, his hands folded on his chest. The room was quiet except for the faint ticking of the clock on the wall. Edward liked mornings like this—calm, still, and full of potential.

He swung his legs over the side of the bed and pushed himself up with a grunt. His knees creaked, but he ignored the discomfort. Pain was nothing new. What bothered him more was the fog in his mind, the haze that had settled over his thoughts in recent years. Frontotemporal dementia had stolen pieces of him—his sharp wit, his precise memory—but it hadn't taken his drive. Not yet.

Edward shuffled to the small dresser in the corner of his room. On top of it sat a row of neatly folded towels, each one the result of his nightly ritual. Folding towels calmed him, gave him a sense of control in a world that often felt chaotic. He picked up the top towel, ran his fingers over the fabric, and then placed it back in the pile. Perfect.

The clock read 5:45 a.m. The rest of Willow Grove Nursing Home was still asleep, but Edward felt restless. He glanced toward the door, an idea forming in his mind. The kitchen—he could reorganize it. Yes, that would keep him busy.

By 6:15 a.m., Edward was in the kitchen. The lights buzzed softly overhead as he opened cabinets and surveyed their contents. Spices, canned goods, utensils—they were all in the wrong places. Who had organized this mess? He muttered under his breath as he began rearranging the shelves, moving items with a precision that belied his shaky hands.

"Salt with salt," he said, placing the shakers in a neat row. "Flour with flour. It's not that hard."

The task absorbed him completely. He didn't hear Maria, the head nurse, enter the kitchen until she cleared her throat.

"Edward," she said, her tone a mix of amusement and exasperation. "What are you doing?"

"Fixing this mess," Edward replied without looking up. "You people don't know how to organize a kitchen."

Maria crossed her arms, watching as Edward carefully aligned a row of jars. She knew better than to scold him. Edward's need for order was one of the ways he coped with his dementia, and as long as he wasn't harming himself or others, she saw no reason to stop him.

"Well, at least you're keeping busy," she said finally. "But let's try to wrap this up before breakfast. The kitchen staff will need their space soon."

Edward nodded, though he didn't stop what he was doing. Maria sighed and left him to his work.

By the time breakfast was served, Edward had finished his reorganization project. He entered the dining room with a sense of accomplishment, a rare smile tugging at the corners of his mouth. He sat down at a table near the center of the room, where Margaret and Linda were already chatting.

"What's got you in such a good mood?" Margaret asked, raising an eyebrow.

"Fixed the kitchen," Edward said simply. "It was a disaster."

Margaret chuckled. "I'm sure the staff appreciated that."

Edward didn't respond. Instead, he turned his attention to his plate of eggs and toast, eating with mechanical precision. He didn't like small talk, not anymore. It was too exhausting, too messy. He preferred tasks—things he could fix, organize, or complete.

After breakfast, Edward made his way to the activity room. A staff member had set up a baking station, complete with bowls, measuring cups, and ingredients. The sight of it made Edward's heart skip. Baking had been his life's work. He'd owned a small bakery in town for over thirty years, a place where people came for fresh bread, pastries, and conversation. Those days felt like a lifetime ago, but the muscle memory was still there, buried beneath the fog.

"Would you like to join us, Edward?" Annie asked, gesturing to the baking station.

Edward hesitated. He didn't like group activities, but something about the setup called to him. He nodded slowly and took a seat.

Today's recipe was chocolate chip cookies, a simple but classic choice. Edward picked up the measuring cup and began scooping flour into a bowl. His movements were deliberate, his hands steady despite the tremors that usually plagued him. As he worked, the fog in his mind seemed to lift, replaced by a clarity he hadn't felt in weeks.

"You're a natural," Annie said, watching him work.

Edward didn't respond. He was too focused on the dough, mixing it with a wooden spoon until it reached the perfect consistency. When it was time to add the chocolate chips, he measured them precisely, refusing to deviate from the recipe.

"You remind me of my father," Linda said from across the table. She was working on her own batch of cookies, though her technique was far less precise. "He used to bake with that same look on his face—so serious."

Edward glanced at her, his expression softening. "Baking isn't just about ingredients," he said. "It's about heart."

The words surprised even him. He hadn't spoken about baking—or anything else, really—with such passion in a long time. For a moment, he felt like himself again.

By lunchtime, the cookies were cooling on a wire rack, filling the room with their sweet aroma. Edward stood back and admired them, a rare sense of pride swelling in his chest. He hadn't baked in years, but today, he'd done something good.

As the residents and staff sampled the cookies, Edward sat quietly, watching their reactions. Linda took a bite and closed her eyes, savoring the flavor. "These are amazing," she said. "You've still got it, Edward."

Margaret nodded in agreement. "You should teach us your secrets."

Edward shook his head. "No secrets. Just practice."

The rest of the day passed in a blur of small tasks and quiet moments. Edward spent part of the afternoon folding towels in his room, the repetitive motion soothing his mind. He thought about the cookies, the smiles they had brought to people's faces. It was a good feeling, one he hadn't experienced in a long time.

As evening fell, Edward joined the other residents in the common room for a movie night. He wasn't particularly interested in the film, but he liked the sense of community. He sat in the back, watching the others more than the screen.

Linda was chatting with Sarah, who was recounting a story about her teaching days. Margaret was knitting, her hands moving with practiced ease. John was scribbling in his crossword puzzle, his brow furrowed in concentration. Edward felt a pang of affection for these people, his unlikely companions in this stage of life.

When the movie ended, Edward returned to his room and sat on the edge of his bed. The kitchen, the cookies, the laughter—it all replayed in his mind. For a moment, the fog lifted again, and he felt the weight of his old self, the man he used to be.

"Not bad," he muttered to himself. "Not bad at all."

He climbed into bed and closed his eyes, the scent of cookies lingering in his memory as he drifted off to sleep.

Chapter 5: Margaret

Margaret stood in the hallway, staring at the bulletin board. She wasn't sure how she had ended up there. The last thing she remembered was stepping out of her room, intending to go to the dining area for breakfast. Now, the colorful photos and announcements pinned to the board held her attention, though she couldn't quite make sense of them.

A small wave of panic began to rise in her chest, but she quickly tamped it down. She hated how disoriented she felt sometimes. The doctors had called it mixed dementia—a combination of Alzheimer's and vascular dementia. Margaret just called it frustrating.

She glanced up and down the hallway, hoping for a familiar face. Her relief was palpable when Annie appeared, carrying a stack of towels toward the laundry room.

"Margaret!" Annie greeted warmly. "Are you lost?"

Margaret hesitated, unsure of how to answer. "I... I think I was going to breakfast," she said finally.

"Well, you're in luck. I was just about to head that way myself," Annie said, setting down the towels. She gently guided Margaret toward the dining room, chatting as they walked. Margaret appreciated Annie's calm presence. It grounded her when the world felt too big and confusing.

By the time Margaret reached the dining room, many of the residents were already seated. Sarah waved her over to a table near the window, where Linda and John were also sitting. Margaret took a seat, smoothing her skirt as she did.

"Good morning," she said, her voice steady, though she felt anything but.

"Good morning, Margaret!" Sarah chirped, her cheerful tone cutting through Margaret's unease. "You're just in time. We were talking about the birds outside."

Margaret followed Sarah's gaze to the garden, where sparrows flitted around the bird feeder. "They're lovely," she said softly, though her mind was elsewhere. She tried to recall what day it was, what month, but the information eluded her.

"Would you like some coffee, Margaret?" Annie asked, appearing beside her.

"Yes, please," Margaret replied. Coffee always helped. Or at least, it used to.

As breakfast progressed, Margaret began to relax. The familiar routine—coffee, toast, polite conversation—gave her a sense of normalcy. She even managed a laugh when Linda mentioned the "parrot" she'd seen that morning.

"You have quite the imagination, Linda," Margaret said with a smile.

"It wasn't my imagination," Linda insisted, though her tone was light. "It was as real as you and me."

Margaret shook her head, amused. It was moments like these that made life at Willow Grove feel less like a nursing home and more like a community.

After breakfast, Margaret decided to visit the activity room. She didn't always participate in the scheduled events, but she enjoyed being around the others. It made her feel less isolated.

Today's activity was a painting session. Linda had already claimed a spot near the window, her brushes and paints laid out before her. Edward was there too, though he seemed more interested in folding towels than painting.

Margaret hesitated at the door, unsure if she should join. Her hands trembled sometimes, and she worried that the others would notice. But Annie spotted her and waved her over.

"Come sit with us, Margaret," Annie said, pulling out a chair. "You don't have to paint if you don't want to. You can just watch."

Margaret nodded and took a seat. She watched as Linda worked on a vibrant painting of a bird—presumably the parrot she'd mentioned earlier. The colors were bold and striking, a stark contrast to the gray fog that often clouded Margaret's mind.

"It's beautiful," Margaret said, leaning closer to get a better look.

"Thank you," Linda replied, her voice tinged with pride. "Do you paint, Margaret?"

"I used to," Margaret said. "A long time ago. But I'm not sure I remember how."

Linda smiled gently. "It's like riding a bike. You never really forget."

Margaret wasn't so sure, but Linda's words stuck with her.

Later in the afternoon, Margaret wandered into the library. It was her favorite room in Willow Grove, filled with rows of books that smelled faintly of old paper and leather bindings. She used to be a librarian, and the sight of the shelves brought her a sense of peace.

She ran her fingers along the spines of the books, pausing occasionally to pull one out and examine the cover. She didn't read as much as she used to—her attention span wasn't what it once was—but she still found comfort in the presence of books.

Annie found her there, flipping through a worn copy of *Little Women*.

"Is that one of your favorites?" Annie asked, sitting down beside her.

"It is," Margaret said, her voice soft. "I used to read it to my daughter when she was little."

Annie's expression warmed. "You must have been a wonderful mother."

"I tried to be," Margaret said, though a shadow crossed her face. She couldn't quite remember her daughter's name. The realization stung, and she quickly closed the book, setting it back on the shelf.

Annie noticed the change in Margaret's demeanor but didn't press her. Instead, she shifted the conversation. "Do you want to help me set up for Iron Chef later? The residents are making chocolate chip cookies today."

Margaret hesitated but nodded. Helping always made her feel better.

By the time the cookies were baking, Margaret felt more at ease. The activity room was filled with the warm, sweet aroma of chocolate, and the residents were chatting animatedly as they waited for the cookies to cool.

Edward, who had taken charge of the baking process, handed Margaret a freshly baked cookie. "Try this," he said, his tone gruff but not unkind.

Margaret took a bite, the chocolate melting on her tongue. For a moment, she felt a flicker of joy—pure and uncomplicated. "It's delicious," she said.

Edward grunted in acknowledgment, clearly pleased with her response.

As evening fell, Margaret found herself back in the common room. The staff had set up a movie night, and residents were gathering around the television. Margaret chose a seat near the back, where she could watch without being too close to the action.

The movie was a lighthearted comedy, and the room filled with laughter as the scenes unfolded. Margaret smiled faintly, though her mind drifted. She thought about the library, about the books she loved but couldn't always remember. She thought about her daughter, whose name danced on the edge of her memory but refused to come into focus.

When the movie ended, Margaret lingered in her seat as the others began to leave. Annie approached her, crouching beside her chair.

"Are you okay, Margaret?" she asked.

Margaret nodded slowly. "I was just thinking. Sometimes, I feel like I'm losing pieces of myself."

Annie placed a reassuring hand on her arm. "Maybe. But the pieces that matter most are still there. I see them every day."

Margaret looked at her, a faint smile tugging at the corners of her mouth. "Thank you, Annie."

"Anytime," Annie said. "Goodnight, Margaret."

"Goodnight," Margaret replied, her voice soft.

Back in her room, Margaret sat on the edge of her bed, staring at the small stack of books on her nightstand. She reached for *Little Women* and opened it to a random page.

The words swam before her eyes, but she didn't mind. Just holding the book was enough.

As she lay down to sleep, the faint smell of chocolate lingered in the air. It reminded her of the cookies, of the warmth of the activity room, of the laughter that had filled the day.

And for a moment, as she drifted off, the fog lifted. She wasn't lost. Not tonight.

Chapter 6: Henry

Henry sat on the edge of his bed, staring at his harmonica as the morning light streamed through his window. The small, silver instrument fit perfectly in his hand, its smooth surface polished to a shine from years of use. It had been his constant companion, his voice when words failed him. Even now, with Parkinson's disease dementia gradually stealing pieces of his memory and control, the harmonica still felt like an extension of himself.

He turned it over in his hands, his fingers trembling slightly. Today was a good day, he decided. His hands were steady enough, his mind clear enough. He raised the harmonica to his lips and blew a soft, trembling note. It filled the quiet room, a mournful, haunting sound that carried the weight of all he couldn't say.

For a moment, Henry closed his eyes and let the music flow. The melody was simple but soulful, a tune he'd played countless times before. It transported him back to the smoky bars and crowded dance halls of his youth, where he'd played for hours on end, losing himself in the rhythm and the roar of applause.

When the tune ended, Henry opened his eyes, his chest tight with longing. Those days were gone, but the music remained.

By the time Henry made it to the dining room for breakfast, most of the residents were already seated. He shuffled in slowly, his movements deliberate, his cane tapping softly against the floor. Annie noticed him immediately and hurried over to help.

"Good morning, Henry," she said with a warm smile. "How are you feeling today?"

"Not bad," Henry replied, his voice gruff but kind. "Hands are working, so I can't complain."

Annie helped him to his usual seat near the center of the room. Sarah was at the table, chatting animatedly with Margaret, and Linda was gazing out the window, lost in thought. Henry nodded a greeting to them all before turning his attention to the plate of scrambled eggs and toast in front of him.

"Did you bring your harmonica today?" Sarah asked, her eyes bright.

Henry tapped the pocket of his cardigan, where the harmonica rested. "Never leave without it."

"You should play for us later," Sarah said. "It always brightens the room."

Henry grunted in acknowledgment, though he wasn't sure if he'd play. The harmonica was deeply personal to him, a connection to his past, and he didn't always feel like sharing it. But Sarah's enthusiasm made him smile.

After breakfast, Henry joined the other residents in the activity room. He preferred to stay on the edges of things, watching rather than participating. Today, the staff had set up a group discussion about favorite memories. Residents took turns sharing stories, and Henry listened quietly, his harmonica clutched tightly in his hand.

When it was his turn to speak, Henry hesitated. He didn't like talking about himself— words often felt clumsy compared to music. But Annie gave him an encouraging nod, and he cleared his throat.

"Used to be a musician," he said simply. His voice was deep and raspy, each word deliberate. "Played the harmonica. Toured with a blues band for years. Good times."

The room was silent for a moment before Sarah chimed in. "That's amazing, Henry! You should play for us now."

Other residents murmured in agreement, their faces lighting up with anticipation. Henry hesitated, his fingers tightening around the harmonica. Then, with a small sigh, he raised it to his lips.

The first notes were soft and tentative, but as the melody grew, so did Henry's confidence. The tune was a classic blues piece, slow and soulful, each note carrying a depth of emotion that words couldn't capture. The room fell silent, the music washing over everyone like a warm wave.

When he finished, the residents broke into applause, their faces filled with admiration. Henry lowered the harmonica, a faint smile tugging at the corners of his mouth.

"Thank you," he said quietly, his voice thick with emotion.

In the afternoon, Henry retreated to the garden. The fresh air and the sound of birds chirping in the trees always soothed him. He found a bench near the edge of the garden and sat down, his harmonica resting on his lap.

As he sat there, a memory surfaced—one of his wife, Mary. She'd loved the garden, spending hours tending to the flowers and humming along to his music. He could almost see her now, kneeling in the dirt with a straw hat on her head and a gentle smile on her face.

"I miss you, Mary," he murmured, his voice barely audible. The ache in his chest was familiar, a constant reminder of the life he'd left behind.

He picked up the harmonica and began to play again, a soft, wistful tune that seemed to rise and fall with the breeze. It was Mary's favorite song, one he'd played for her on their wedding day. As the music filled the garden, Henry felt a sense of peace, as though Mary were sitting beside him, listening.

By evening, Henry was back in the common room for a movie night. He chose a seat near the back, where he could watch without feeling too exposed. The room was lively, filled with laughter and conversation, but Henry remained quiet, content to observe.

The movie was a lighthearted comedy, and the residents laughed at all the right moments. Henry found himself smiling too, though his mind was only half on the screen. He watched the others—Sarah, Linda, Edward, Margaret—and felt a strange sense of belonging.

When the movie ended, Annie approached him as the other residents began to leave.

"Thank you for playing earlier," she said, her smile warm. "You made everyone's day."

Henry shrugged, though he felt a flicker of pride. "It's just music."

"It's more than that," Annie said. "It's a gift."

Henry nodded, his gaze dropping to the harmonica in his hand. "Guess it is."

Later that night, as Henry lay in bed, he stared at the harmonica on his nightstand. The day had been a good one, filled with moments of connection and clarity. He'd played his music, shared a piece of himself, and been reminded of the joy it could bring to others.

As he closed his eyes, he thought of Mary and the garden, of smoky bars and roaring applause, of the life he'd lived and the music that still remained. And with that thought, he drifted off to sleep, a faint smile on his lips.

Chapter 7: Emily

Emily sat at the edge of her bed, staring at her reflection in the small mirror on her dresser. Her fingers traced the curve of her cheek, brushing against the faint lines that had begun to deepen over the years. Her body felt foreign to her now, uncooperative and unpredictable, a cruel betrayal by Huntington's disease. Her movements were jerky, involuntary twitches disrupting what should have been graceful motions. But her spirit? Her spirit still held onto the echoes of the vibrant woman she once was.

"I'm still here," she whispered, as if trying to convince herself.

The early morning light filtered through the curtains, illuminating the framed photos on her dresser. One picture, in particular, drew her gaze—a black-and-white snapshot of her dancing with her father at a wedding. She was just a teenager then, spinning in a polka-dotted dress, her hair bouncing with every turn.

She closed her eyes and swayed slightly, imagining the music. The memory was sharp, a bright contrast to the foggy haze that often clouded her mind. She could hear her father's voice, feel his steady hands guiding her across the floor.

A knock at the door startled her. She turned sharply, her movements exaggerated by the involuntary jerks of her condition. Annie peeked in, her face bright with a warm smile.

"Good morning, Emily. Ready for breakfast?"

Emily nodded, the tension in her shoulders easing. Annie always had a way of grounding her, making the chaos inside her body feel manageable.

By the time Emily reached the dining room, most of the residents were already seated. She spotted Linda and Margaret at a table near the window, deep in conversation. Henry sat at another table, his harmonica resting in his lap as he sipped his coffee. Emily made her way to a corner table, preferring a quieter spot.

"Good morning, Emily," Sarah called from across the room, her voice chipper. "Come sit with us!"

Emily hesitated. She liked Sarah's energy—it was infectious—but she wasn't sure she had the stamina for a full breakfast conversation. Before she could decide, Annie appeared beside her, gently guiding her to a seat.

"Why don't you join Sarah and the others today?" Annie suggested. "I think they'd love to have you."

Emily sighed but allowed herself to be led to Sarah's table. As soon as she sat down, Sarah launched into a story about the birds she'd seen outside that morning, her hands gesturing animatedly. Emily listened quietly, a faint smile tugging at her lips. It was nice to feel included, even if she didn't always have the energy to contribute.

After breakfast, the staff had planned a light exercise class in the activity room. Emily considered skipping it—her body didn't always cooperate with structured movement—but Annie encouraged her to join.

"It's not about doing it perfectly," Annie said. "It's about moving and having fun."

Emily reluctantly agreed and found herself standing in a loose circle with the other residents. The instructor, a cheerful woman named Kayla, led them through gentle stretches and simple movements. Emily tried to follow along, but her body rebelled, her arms jerking in sharp, uncoordinated motions.

"Don't worry about keeping up," Kayla said, her tone encouraging. "Just do what feels good."

Emily glanced around the room, noticing that everyone was focused on their own movements. No one seemed to be watching her, and that realization eased her anxiety. She swayed to the music playing softly in the background, letting her body move however it wanted. The jerks and twitches didn't matter here. She was dancing in her own way.

"You look beautiful," Sarah said from across the circle, her voice warm.

Emily felt her cheeks flush. She hadn't been called beautiful in years, not since the symptoms of her disease had become impossible to hide. But in that moment, she believed it.

After the exercise class, Emily wandered into the garden. The crisp autumn air was invigorating, and the sight of the flowers still in bloom brought her a sense of peace. She walked slowly along the stone path, her movements uneven but determined.

She stopped by a wooden bench and sat down, her gaze drifting to the bird feeder hanging from a nearby tree. A small sparrow darted in and out, pecking at the seeds. Emily smiled, reminded of the birds Sarah had mentioned at breakfast.

A memory surfaced—dancing in the garden at her cousin's wedding. The music had been loud and lively, the laughter infectious. She had danced barefoot on the grass, her dress swirling around her as the sun set behind the trees.

She closed her eyes and hummed a few bars of the song she'd danced to that evening. Her foot tapped against the ground, keeping time with the rhythm in her mind. For a moment, she felt like that carefree girl again, the one who danced as though the world were hers.

By the afternoon, the residents had gathered in the activity room for Iron Chef. Today's challenge was making chocolate chip cookies, and Emily found herself drawn to the familiar activity. Baking had always been a source of comfort for her, a way to create something tangible and satisfying.

Annie handed her a bowl and a wooden spoon. "Let's see what you've got, Emily."

Emily smiled, her hands gripping the spoon tightly as she began to mix the dough. The movements were clumsy, her jerks and twitches making the process messier than she'd intended, but Annie didn't seem to mind.

"You're doing great," Annie said, wiping a bit of flour from Emily's cheek.

Emily laughed, a sound she hadn't heard from herself in days. She kept mixing, the familiar rhythm of baking easing her mind. When the cookies went into the oven, she felt a swell of pride. She had created something—something good.

That evening, as the residents gathered for movie night, Emily chose a seat near the front. The day had left her feeling lighter, more connected to the others. The movie—a lighthearted comedy—brought plenty of laughter, and Emily found herself joining in, her laughter mingling with the rest.

When the movie ended, Annie approached her with a warm smile. "You did a lot today, Emily. I'm proud of you."

Emily nodded, her eyes glistening. "It felt good," she admitted.

"Good," Annie said. "You deserve to feel good."

Back in her room, Emily sat on the edge of her bed, staring at the photo of her and her father on the dresser. She reached for it, running her fingers over the glass.

"I danced today," she whispered. "Not like I used to, but I danced."

As she climbed into bed, she felt a sense of peace. The day had been filled with small victories—dancing, baking, laughing. They were moments of joy that reminded her she was still herself, even as her body betrayed her.

And with that thought, Emily drifted off to sleep, her father's voice echoing in her mind: "Keep dancing, sweetheart. Always keep dancing."

Chapter 7: Emily

Emily sat at the edge of her bed, staring at her reflection in the small mirror on her dresser. Her fingers traced the curve of her cheek, brushing against the faint lines that had begun to deepen over the years. Her body felt foreign to her now, uncooperative and unpredictable, a cruel betrayal by Huntington's disease. Her movements were jerky, involuntary twitches disrupting what should have been graceful motions. But her spirit? Her spirit still held onto the echoes of the vibrant woman she once was.

"I'm still here," she whispered, as if trying to convince herself.

The early morning light filtered through the curtains, illuminating the framed photos on her dresser. One picture, in particular, drew her gaze—a black-and-white snapshot of her dancing with her father at a wedding. She was just a teenager then, spinning in a polka-dotted dress, her hair bouncing with every turn.

She closed her eyes and swayed slightly, imagining the music. The memory was sharp, a bright contrast to the foggy haze that often clouded her mind. She could hear her father's voice, feel his steady hands guiding her across the floor.

A knock at the door startled her. She turned sharply, her movements exaggerated by the involuntary jerks of her condition. Annie peeked in, her face bright with a warm smile.

"Good morning, Emily. Ready for breakfast?"

Emily nodded, the tension in her shoulders easing. Annie always had a way of grounding her, making the chaos inside her body feel manageable.

By the time Emily reached the dining room, most of the residents were already seated. She spotted Linda and Margaret at a table near the window, deep in conversation. Henry sat at another table, his harmonica resting in his lap as he sipped his coffee. Emily made her way to a corner table, preferring a quieter spot.

"Good morning, Emily," Sarah called from across the room, her voice chipper. "Come sit with us!"

Emily hesitated. She liked Sarah's energy—it was infectious—but she wasn't sure she had the stamina for a full breakfast conversation. Before she could decide, Annie appeared beside her, gently guiding her to a seat.

"Why don't you join Sarah and the others today?" Annie suggested. "I think they'd love to have you."

Emily sighed but allowed herself to be led to Sarah's table. As soon as she sat down, Sarah launched into a story about the birds she'd seen outside that morning, her hands gesturing animatedly. Emily listened quietly, a faint smile tugging at her lips. It was nice to feel included, even if she didn't always have the energy to contribute.

After breakfast, the staff had planned a light exercise class in the activity room. Emily considered skipping it—her body didn't always cooperate with structured movement—but Annie encouraged her to join.

"It's not about doing it perfectly," Annie said. "It's about moving and having fun."

Emily reluctantly agreed and found herself standing in a loose circle with the other residents. The instructor, a cheerful woman named Kayla, led them through gentle stretches and simple movements. Emily tried to follow along, but her body rebelled, her arms jerking in sharp, uncoordinated motions.

"Don't worry about keeping up," Kayla said, her tone encouraging. "Just do what feels good."

Emily glanced around the room, noticing that everyone was focused on their own movements. No one seemed to be watching her, and that realization eased her anxiety. She swayed to the music playing softly in the background, letting her body move however it wanted. The jerks and twitches didn't matter here. She was dancing in her own way.

"You look beautiful," Sarah said from across the circle, her voice warm.

Emily felt her cheeks flush. She hadn't been called beautiful in years, not since the symptoms of her disease had become impossible to hide. But in that moment, she believed it.

After the exercise class, Emily wandered into the garden. The crisp autumn air was invigorating, and the sight of the flowers still in bloom brought her a sense of peace. She walked slowly along the stone path, her movements uneven but determined.

She stopped by a wooden bench and sat down, her gaze drifting to the bird feeder hanging from a nearby tree. A small sparrow darted in and out, pecking at the seeds. Emily smiled, reminded of the birds Sarah had mentioned at breakfast.

A memory surfaced—dancing in the garden at her cousin's wedding. The music had been loud and lively, the laughter infectious. She had danced barefoot on the grass, her dress swirling around her as the sun set behind the trees.

She closed her eyes and hummed a few bars of the song she'd danced to that evening. Her foot tapped against the ground, keeping time with the rhythm in her mind. For a moment, she felt like that carefree girl again, the one who danced as though the world were hers.

By the afternoon, the residents had gathered in the activity room for Iron Chef. Today's challenge was making chocolate chip cookies, and Emily found herself drawn to the familiar activity. Baking had always been a source of comfort for her, a way to create something tangible and satisfying.

Annie handed her a bowl and a wooden spoon. "Let's see what you've got, Emily."

Emily smiled, her hands gripping the spoon tightly as she began to mix the dough. The movements were clumsy, her jerks and twitches making the process messier than she'd intended, but Annie didn't seem to mind.

"You're doing great," Annie said, wiping a bit of flour from Emily's cheek.

Emily laughed, a sound she hadn't heard from herself in days. She kept mixing, the familiar rhythm of baking easing her mind. When the cookies went into the oven, she felt a swell of pride. She had created something—something good.

That evening, as the residents gathered for movie night, Emily chose a seat near the front. The day had left her feeling lighter, more connected to the others. The movie—a lighthearted comedy—brought plenty of laughter, and Emily found herself joining in, her laughter mingling with the rest.

When the movie ended, Annie approached her with a warm smile. "You did a lot today, Emily. I'm proud of you."

Emily nodded, her eyes glistening. "It felt good," she admitted.

"Good," Annie said. "You deserve to feel good."

Back in her room, Emily sat on the edge of her bed, staring at the photo of her and her father on the dresser. She reached for it, running her fingers over the glass.

"I danced today," she whispered. "Not like I used to, but I danced."

As she climbed into bed, she felt a sense of peace. The day had been filled with small victories—dancing, baking, laughing. They were moments of joy that reminded her she was still herself, even as her body betrayed her.

And with that thought, Emily drifted off to sleep, her father's voice echoing in her mind: "Keep dancing, sweetheart. Always keep dancing."

Chapter 8: Robert

Robert sat in his chair by the window, staring at the tree just outside. The leaves were a fiery mix of orange and gold, their colors vibrant against the pale autumn sky. He wanted to hold onto the image, to burn it into his memory, but he knew it wouldn't last. The memories never did anymore. Creutzfeldt-Jakob disease had taken so much from him already—his ability to speak fluently, his coordination, his independence—and it was determined to take more.

His room was quiet except for the faint ticking of the clock on the wall. The silence was a stark contrast to the noise that often filled his mind. Robert sometimes imagined it as static, like an old radio unable to tune into the right station. Today, though, the static was softer, and he was grateful for the reprieve.

"Robert?" A familiar voice broke the silence. Annie stood in the doorway, her kind eyes scanning his face. "How are you this morning?"

He nodded slowly, his movements deliberate. Words felt too heavy to form, so he simply pointed to the tree outside.

"The leaves are beautiful, aren't they?" Annie said, stepping closer. "Would you like to go outside and see them up close?"

Robert nodded again, his chest tightening with gratitude. Annie always seemed to know what he needed, even when he couldn't say it.

A few minutes later, Robert was bundled in a thick sweater, sitting in his wheelchair as Annie pushed him toward the garden. The crisp air hit his face, refreshing and sharp, and he inhaled deeply. The scent of damp earth and fallen leaves filled his senses, grounding him in the moment.

Annie parked the wheelchair near the tree, positioning him so he could see the leaves up close. Robert reached out a trembling hand, his fingers brushing against the rough bark of the trunk. It was solid, unchanging, a stark contrast to the fragility he felt within himself.

"I thought you might like this," Annie said, crouching beside him. She held out a small notebook and a pen. "Would you like to write something down? Maybe a memory?"

Robert stared at the notebook for a long moment before taking it. His handwriting had grown shaky and uneven, but the act of writing still brought him comfort. He opened the notebook to a blank page and pressed the pen to the paper.

Mary loved the fall.

The letters were jagged, some barely legible, but Annie didn't seem to mind. She watched quietly as he wrote, her presence steady and reassuring.

She said it was the season of change. She was right.

When he finished, he set the pen down, his hand trembling from the effort. Annie picked up the notebook and read the words aloud, her voice soft.

"She sounds like a wise woman," Annie said, smiling.

Robert nodded, his throat tight. Mary had been everything to him—his wife, his anchor, his greatest love. Losing her had been like losing a part of himself, and now, with his disease progressing, he feared losing the memories of her too.

Back inside, Robert spent the morning in the activity room. The other residents were gathered for a discussion about their favorite seasons, but Robert stayed on the edges of the group, his notebook resting on his lap. He flipped through the pages, rereading the words he'd written in the past weeks.

Most of the entries were simple—short phrases or fragmented thoughts—but they were his lifeline. They reminded him of who he was, who he'd been, and the people he'd loved.

"Robert," Annie said, approaching him with a gentle smile. "Would you like to share something with the group?"

He hesitated. Speaking was difficult, and he didn't like the way his voice sounded now—halting, unsteady. But Annie's encouragement gave him courage. He handed her the notebook, tapping the page he'd written earlier.

Annie read the words aloud: "Mary loved the fall. She said it was the season of change. She was right."

The room fell silent for a moment, the weight of the words settling over the group. Then Sarah spoke up, her voice bright.

"That's beautiful, Robert," she said. "You must have loved her very much."

Robert nodded, his eyes glistening. He felt a swell of gratitude toward Annie for giving his words a voice, for making him feel seen.

In the afternoon, Robert joined the others in the activity room for Iron Chef. He wasn't much of a cook—Mary had always handled that—but he enjoyed watching the process. Today's recipe was chocolate chip cookies, and the room buzzed with energy as the residents measured, mixed, and baked.

Edward, ever precise, took charge of one station, while Linda added her artistic flair to another. Robert sat quietly, observing the chaos with a faint smile. He didn't mind being on the sidelines; it gave him a chance to soak in the moment.

Annie appeared beside him, holding a small bowl of dough. "Would you like to help shape the cookies?" she asked.

Robert hesitated, his hands trembling in his lap. But Annie's gentle encouragement gave him the confidence to try. She placed a spoon in his hand and guided it to the dough. Together, they shaped small mounds onto the baking sheet, each one imperfect but uniquely theirs.

When the cookies came out of the oven, Robert felt a small sense of pride. He hadn't done much, but he'd been part of it, part of something.

By evening, Robert was back in his room, the notebook open on his lap. The day had been full—perhaps too full—but it had also been good. He picked up the pen and wrote another entry:

I shaped cookies today. They weren't perfect, but they were mine.

He stared at the words for a long time, letting their meaning sink in. It wasn't just about the cookies. It was about holding onto the small victories, the moments that made him feel like himself again.

Annie knocked softly on the door, peeking in. "Goodnight, Robert. Do you need anything before bed?"

Robert shook his head and gestured to the notebook, a silent thank you for her suggestion earlier. Annie smiled and stepped inside, placing a hand on his shoulder.

"You did great today, Robert," she said. "I'm proud of you."

Her words warmed him, and for the first time in a long while, he believed them.

That night, as Robert lay in bed, he stared at the notebook on his nightstand. The memories inside it were imperfect, fragmented, but they were his. And as he closed his eyes, he felt a sense of peace.

Because even as his disease tried to take everything from him, he still had his words. And that was enough.

Chapter 9: Mildred

Mildred's day began with a careful ritual. She sat on the edge of her bed, her feet flat against the floor, and ran her fingers through her thinning silver hair. Her mirror reflected a woman who still held herself with dignity, despite the challenges of her condition. Normal Pressure Hydrocephalus had left her movements hesitant, her gait unsteady, and her memory unreliable. But Mildred refused to let it define her.

Her room was tidy, every item in its place—a habit she'd carried from her days as a nurse. She reached for the small brooch on her dresser, a simple gold pin in the shape of a dove. She fastened it to the lapel of her cardigan, taking comfort in its familiar weight.

"I'm ready," she whispered to herself, though her voice wavered.

There was a knock at the door, and Annie stepped in, her bright smile lighting up the room.

"Good morning, Mildred," Annie said, her voice warm. "How are you feeling today?"

"Better, I think," Mildred replied. "Steady enough to make it to breakfast."

"That's what I like to hear," Annie said, offering her arm. "Shall we?"

Mildred nodded and stood slowly, leaning on Annie as they made their way to the dining room. Each step felt deliberate, a reminder of the effort it took to stay upright. But Mildred took pride in her perseverance. She had always been strong, and she wasn't about to stop now.

The dining room buzzed with the usual morning energy. Sarah greeted Mildred with a cheerful wave, while Linda and Margaret chatted near the window. Mildred took her seat at a table near the center of the room, the dove brooch catching the light.

"Good morning, ladies," she said, her voice calm and composed.

"Good morning, Mildred!" Sarah said, her voice bright. "How are you today?"

"Steady enough," Mildred replied with a small smile. "And you?"

"Wonderful," Sarah said, launching into a story about the birds outside. Mildred listened politely, her hands folded neatly in her lap. She admired Sarah's enthusiasm, even if she didn't always have the energy to match it.

As breakfast was served, Mildred focused on the simple act of eating. The soft clinking of cutlery against plates was a comforting rhythm, grounding her in the present. She sipped her coffee slowly, savoring its warmth.

After breakfast, Mildred decided to join the morning walking group. The idea both excited and intimidated her. Walking had once been second nature, but now it required careful attention, each step a deliberate act of balance and coordination.

"You've got this," Annie said as she helped Mildred into her walking shoes. "Just take it slow. There's no rush."

Mildred nodded, gripping her cane tightly as the group made their way outside. The garden path was lined with colorful flowers, their petals bright against the autumn leaves. The air was crisp, carrying the faint scent of damp earth.

The other residents moved ahead, their laughter drifting back to her. Mildred focused on the ground beneath her feet, the steady tap of her cane against the stone path. One step, then another. She paused by a bench, her breath coming in short bursts.

"You're doing great," Annie said, her voice encouraging. "Do you want to rest for a bit?"

"No," Mildred said firmly. "I can keep going."

Annie smiled, her admiration evident. Mildred's determination was one of her most defining traits, a testament to the strength she carried from her years as a nurse.

By the time the group completed the circuit, Mildred felt both exhausted and triumphant. She sank onto a bench, her chest heaving with effort, but her face lit with a rare smile.

"I did it," she said, her voice barely above a whisper.

"You did," Annie agreed. "I'm proud of you."

In the afternoon, Mildred joined the others in the activity room for Iron Chef. She wasn't much of a baker, but she enjoyed being part of the group. The camaraderie reminded her of her days working in a bustling hospital, surrounded by colleagues who shared her dedication.

Edward took charge of the cookie-making process, his precision evident in every step. Mildred found herself impressed by his focus, even as her own hands trembled slightly while measuring the flour.

"Here, let me help," Annie said, steadying the measuring cup.

Mildred nodded gratefully, though she felt a pang of frustration at her body's limitations. But as the cookies baked, filling the room with their warm, sweet aroma, she felt a sense of accomplishment. She had contributed, however small her role might have been.

When the cookies were ready, Mildred took a bite, the chocolate melting on her tongue. It was a simple pleasure, but it filled her with a quiet joy.

As evening fell, Mildred returned to her room. The day had been full, and her body ached from the effort of walking and baking. But it was a good ache, one that reminded her of what she was still capable of.

She sat by the window, watching the sky fade from gold to deep indigo. The dove brooch on her cardigan glinted faintly in the dim light. She reached up and touched it, her fingers tracing its smooth surface.

The brooch had been a gift from one of her patients many years ago, a token of gratitude for the care she had provided. It was a reminder of who she was—a healer, a caregiver, a woman who had dedicated her life to helping others.

As she climbed into bed, Mildred felt a sense of peace. The day had been challenging, but it had also been full of moments that reminded her of her strength. She closed her eyes, the image of the garden path and the sound of her cane tapping against the stones replaying in her mind.

And as sleep claimed her, Mildred whispered to herself: "I'm still here."

Chapter 10: Frank

Frank woke up with a start, his dream evaporating into the morning light like steam from a cup of coffee. He rubbed his eyes and sat up in bed, his mind spinning with a jumble of images that didn't quite make sense. A crowded bar, laughter echoing against the walls, the clinking of glasses—it all felt so vivid, yet so far away. That was the thing about Wernicke-Korsakoff Syndrome: his memories came and went as they pleased, like uninvited guests at a party.

He stretched, wincing as his back protested the movement, and glanced at the clock on the nightstand. It was later than he'd intended to get up, but time didn't mean much to him these days. Every day was a new story, and Frank was nothing if not a storyteller.

"Another day, another adventure," he muttered, swinging his legs over the side of the bed. He reached for the flannel shirt draped over the chair and pulled it on, the soft fabric a comforting reminder of the past—though exactly what past, he couldn't always say.

When Frank shuffled into the dining room, the usual breakfast crowd was already gathered. Sarah waved him over with a bright smile, and he joined her table, where Linda and Margaret were chatting quietly.

"Good morning, Frank," Sarah said cheerfully. "Sleep well?"

"Like a baby," Frank replied with a grin. "Though I think I dreamed I was in Paris last night. Or maybe it was Las Vegas. Hard to tell with all the lights."

"Paris, huh?" Sarah said, intrigued. "What were you doing there?"

"Oh, you know," Frank said, leaning back in his chair. "Sipping wine on the Seine, chatting with artists about the meaning of life. They all said I had the best ideas they'd ever heard."

Linda chuckled, shaking her head. "And what were those ideas, Frank?"

Frank hesitated, his grin faltering for just a moment. He didn't have an answer—his stories were always full of holes—but he recovered quickly.

"Trade secrets, my dear," he said with a wink. "Can't go giving away all my brilliance for free."

The table laughed, and Frank's chest swelled with pride. He might not remember much these days, but he could still tell a good story.

After breakfast, Frank wandered into the activity room, where Annie was setting up for the morning's group discussion. A colorful poster on the wall read, "Share Your Favorite Memory."

Frank stared at the poster, his brow furrowing. Favorite memory? That was a tough one. His memories were like a deck of cards, shuffled out of order and missing a few key pieces.

"Frank, would you like to join us?" Annie asked, her voice kind.

He hesitated but nodded. He took a seat in the circle of chairs, where the other residents were already sharing their stories. Sarah talked about her days as a teacher, and Margaret recounted a summer spent by the lake with her family. When it was Frank's turn, he cleared his throat, leaning forward in his chair.

"Well," he began, "there was this one time I was in a little jazz club in New Orleans. The band was playing the blues, and the whole room was alive with energy. I got up on stage and sang with them—completely spur of the moment, mind you—and the crowd went wild. They even asked me to come back the next night."

The group listened intently, their faces lighting up with admiration. Annie smiled, though she knew the story wasn't entirely true. Still, she didn't interrupt. For Frank, storytelling was a way to connect, to fill the gaps in his memory with something meaningful.

"What did you sing?" Henry asked from the back of the room, his harmonica resting on his lap.

Frank paused, his mind scrambling for an answer. "Oh, you know, one of those classics. 'Summertime,' maybe. Or was it 'Mack the Knife'? Doesn't matter—it brought the house down."

The group chuckled, and Frank relaxed. He might not remember the details, but he remembered the feeling. That was enough.

In the afternoon, Frank joined the others in the activity room for Iron Chef. The residents were making chocolate chip cookies, and Frank was more than happy to jump in. He donned an apron and grabbed a mixing bowl, his hands surprisingly steady as he measured out ingredients.

"You sure you've done this before?" Edward asked from across the table, his tone skeptical.

"Are you kidding?" Frank said with a laugh. "I used to be a pastry chef. Worked in the finest kitchens in New York City."

Edward raised an eyebrow but didn't press further. Frank grinned to himself, enjoying the little embellishment. The truth didn't matter as much as the story.

As the cookies baked, Frank regaled the group with more tales—some real, most invented. He talked about traveling the world, meeting famous people, and narrowly escaping a lion on safari. The room filled with laughter, the scent of baking cookies mingling with the warmth of shared joy.

Annie watched from the corner, her heart swelling. Frank's stories might not always be accurate, but they brought people together. That was a gift.

By evening, Frank was back in the common room for movie night. The day's activities had left him pleasantly tired, but he still had enough energy to join the group. He chose a seat near the middle, where he could chat with Sarah and Linda.

The movie—a lighthearted comedy—brought plenty of laughter, and Frank found himself caught up in the humor. He didn't always follow the plot, but the energy in the room was infectious.

When the movie ended, Annie approached him with a warm smile. "Did you enjoy it, Frank?"

"Of course," he said, though he couldn't quite remember the ending. "You know, I met the lead actor once. Great guy. Told me I should be in the movies."

Annie chuckled, her eyes twinkling. "I don't doubt it."

Later that night, Frank sat in his room, staring at the small photo on his nightstand. It was an old picture of him in his younger days, standing behind the bar he used to manage. He couldn't remember the name of the bar, or even where it had been, but the smile on his face told him it had been a good time.

He climbed into bed, pulling the blanket up to his chin. His mind was quieter now, the static less insistent. The day had been full of laughter and connection, and for that, he was grateful.

As he drifted off to sleep, Frank whispered to himself, "Another good story."

Chapter 11: Patricia

Patricia sat at her desk, staring at a photo album she hadn't opened in years. Her hands hovered over the cover, hesitant to turn the pages. She loved these photos—her travels, her family, her life—but Posterior Cortical Atrophy had made them harder to see. The once-clear images had become blurry, distorted, as if viewed through frosted glass.

With a deep breath, she opened the album and squinted at the first page. The photo was of her and her husband, Anthony, standing on a beach. She could barely make out the waves in the background, and their faces were hazy, but she remembered the day vividly. It was their honeymoon, a warm summer afternoon when the world had felt endless and bright.

"Anthony always said I looked like a movie star in this photo," she murmured to herself, tracing the outline of her younger self.

A knock at the door interrupted her thoughts, and Annie peeked in, her cheerful smile brightening the dim room.

"Good morning, Patricia," Annie said. "How are you today?"

"Trying to remember," Patricia replied, gesturing to the album. "But it's harder than it used to be."

Annie walked over and glanced at the open page. "That's a lovely photo. Where was it taken?"

"Miami Beach," Patricia said, her voice soft. "Our honeymoon."

Annie sat beside her, tilting the album toward the light. "Tell me about it."

For a moment, Patricia hesitated. The details were slippery, like trying to hold water in her hands. But as she spoke, fragments came together—sunburned shoulders, laughter carried on the breeze, the smell of saltwater and sunscreen. Annie listened patiently, her presence steady and reassuring.

By the time Patricia arrived in the dining room for breakfast, the usual chatter filled the air. She chose a seat near the window, where the light was brightest. Sarah and Margaret were already there, talking about the garden.

"Good morning, Patricia," Sarah said warmly. "Did you see the flowers today? They're so bright and colorful."

"I didn't," Patricia admitted. "But I'd like to."

"We'll have to go after breakfast," Sarah said, her enthusiasm infectious. "You'll love it."

Patricia smiled faintly, though the thought of walking outside made her nervous. Depth perception had become a challenge, and uneven surfaces felt treacherous. Still, Sarah's excitement was hard to resist.

As breakfast progressed, Patricia found herself listening more than speaking. The faces around her were familiar, though sometimes she struggled to match names with them. But the comfort of their presence—their voices, their laughter—made her feel less alone.

After breakfast, Patricia joined the others in the activity room for an art session. Linda was already seated near the window, her paints spread out before her. Patricia hesitated at the doorway, unsure if she could contribute.

"Come sit with me," Linda called, waving her over. "We can paint together."

Patricia nodded and took a seat beside her. Annie placed a blank canvas and a palette of paints in front of her, encouraging her to give it a try.

"I don't know if I can," Patricia admitted, her voice low. "Everything looks... off."

"It doesn't have to be perfect," Annie said gently. "Just paint what you feel."

Patricia picked up a brush and dipped it into the blue paint. The first stroke was hesitant, uneven, but she pressed on. As the brush moved across the canvas, she found herself focusing less on the details and more on the colors—the way they blended, the way they flowed. She painted a beach, or at least her memory of one, with soft waves and a bright horizon.

"That's beautiful," Linda said, glancing at her work. "Is it a memory?"

"Yes," Patricia said softly. "A beach from long ago."

The words stirred something in her—a bittersweet ache for the things she could no longer see clearly, but also a gratitude for the things she could still feel.

In the afternoon, Patricia joined Sarah and Annie for a walk in the garden. The sun was warm on her face, and the scent of flowers filled the air. Patricia walked slowly, her steps careful as she navigated the uneven path.

"Look at those roses," Sarah said, pointing to a cluster of red blooms. "Aren't they stunning?"

Patricia squinted, trying to bring the flowers into focus. They were blurry, their edges soft and indistinct, but the color was vibrant, bold.

"They're beautiful," she said, her voice tinged with wonder. "I wish I could see them better."

Sarah took her hand, giving it a gentle squeeze. "You don't have to see everything to feel it, Patricia. Sometimes, just being here is enough."

Patricia nodded, her chest tightening with emotion. She closed her eyes and let the warmth of the sun, the scent of the flowers, and the sound of Sarah's voice wash over her. For a moment, she felt whole.

That evening, Patricia sat in the common room with the other residents for movie night. The screen was too far for her to see clearly, but she didn't mind. The sound of laughter, the familiar rhythm of dialogue, was enough.

Annie sat beside her, noticing the faint smile on Patricia's face. "Are you enjoying it?" she asked.

"I am," Patricia said. "Even if I can't see it all, I can still feel it."

Annie placed a hand on her arm. "You're amazing, Patricia. You find beauty even in the blur."

Patricia's smile grew. "I've had a lot of practice."

Back in her room, Patricia sat at her desk, the photo album open once again. She ran her fingers over the page, tracing the outlines of the photos. Her vision might be fading, but her heart held onto the memories, even if they were imperfect.

As she climbed into bed, she whispered a silent prayer of gratitude—for the colors, the voices, the moments that still found their way to her.

And as she drifted off to sleep, she dreamed of the beach, the sun on her skin, and the sound of Anthony's laughter carried on the wind.

Chapter 12: Carlos

Carlos stared at the ceiling of his room, the morning sunlight casting long shadows across the walls. The air felt heavy today, and so did his thoughts. Living with HIV-Associated Neurocognitive Disorder had made every day a puzzle he had to piece together—sometimes successfully, often not. His mind felt like a radio station stuck between signals, snippets of clarity interrupted by static.

He turned his head to look at the photo on his bedside table. It was a picture of him in his twenties, grinning widely with his arm slung around his best friend, Mateo. The two of them had been inseparable, causing chaos and cracking jokes like they owned the world.

"Wonder what Mateo would think of me now," Carlos muttered. The thought stung, but he pushed it aside. He had learned to live with these feelings, even if they never quite went away.

A knock on the door broke his reverie. Annie stepped in, her smile as bright as ever.

"Good morning, Carlos," she said. "Ready for breakfast?"

Carlos nodded, though he didn't feel particularly hungry. Annie's presence was always comforting, and he didn't want to let her down.

The dining room was alive with conversation, the usual morning energy buzzing around him. Carlos took his seat near the middle of the room, close enough to hear the chatter but far enough to avoid being the center of attention. He preferred observing to participating.

"Good morning, Carlos," Sarah said, waving from across the table. "You look handsome today."

Carlos chuckled, adjusting his sweater. "Just trying to keep up with you, Sarah."

She laughed, her warmth cutting through the fog in his mind. Carlos appreciated Sarah's friendliness, even on days when he struggled to respond in kind.

As breakfast was served, Carlos focused on the simple act of eating. The toast was warm, the eggs fluffy, but his mind wandered to fragments of memories—Sunday mornings with his mother making tortillas, the smell of fresh coffee filling their small kitchen. He closed his eyes for a moment, savoring the ghost of the memory.

After breakfast, Annie suggested Carlos join the morning's group discussion. The theme was "Beliefs That Shape Us," an opportunity for the residents to share their thoughts and ideas.

Carlos hesitated. He wasn't sure he wanted to speak, but the idea intrigued him. He followed Annie to the activity room, where the chairs were arranged in a circle. Residents like Sarah and Margaret were already there, chatting softly.

Annie opened the discussion by inviting each person to share something they believed in. Sarah spoke about the power of kindness, and Linda shared her love for art as a way to express emotions. When it was Carlos's turn, he felt a lump form in his throat.

"I... I believe in second chances," he said finally, his voice low but steady. "Life doesn't always go the way you plan, but sometimes, you get another shot."

The group nodded, their faces thoughtful. Carlos relaxed, the weight of his words lifting some of the heaviness he'd felt earlier. Annie gave him an encouraging smile, and for a moment, he felt seen.

In the afternoon, Carlos joined the others in the activity room for Iron Chef. Baking wasn't something he'd done much of, but he liked the idea of creating something from scratch. Edward, ever meticulous, handed him a measuring cup and pointed to the flour.

"Don't mess it up," Edward said with a smirk.

Carlos laughed, the sound surprising even himself. "No promises," he replied, scooping the flour into a bowl.

As the residents worked, the room filled with the sound of laughter and the sweet aroma of chocolate chip cookies baking in the oven. Carlos found himself enjoying the process, the act of mixing and measuring grounding him in the present.

When the cookies were done, Annie handed him one to try. The chocolate melted on his tongue, and he couldn't help but smile.

"These are good," he said, his voice filled with genuine delight.

"You helped make them," Annie reminded him.

Carlos nodded, a small flicker of pride warming his chest. It wasn't much, but it was something. And in moments like these, something was enough.

As evening fell, Carlos joined the others for movie night. He chose a seat near the back, where he could watch the screen without feeling too exposed. The movie—a lighthearted comedy—brought plenty of laughter, and Carlos found himself chuckling along with the rest.

When the movie ended, Annie approached him with a question. "Carlos, did you like it?"

"I did," he said, though he couldn't remember much of the plot. "It was... funny."

Annie nodded, her smile soft. "I'm glad."

Back in his room, Carlos sat on the edge of his bed, the photo of him and Mateo in his hands. He stared at their younger selves, the joy and confidence radiating from their faces. He thought about second chances, about the life he was still trying to piece together.

Before climbing into bed, he placed the photo back on the nightstand and whispered to it, "I'm still here, Mateo. Still trying."

As he drifted off to sleep, the echoes of laughter and the warmth of cookies filled his mind, a reminder that even in the static, moments of clarity and connection were still possible.

Chapter 13: Evening Glow

The sun dipped below the horizon, casting long, golden shadows across Willow Grove Nursing Home. The residents gathered in the common room, drawn together by the promise of music, laughter, and connection. Tonight wasn't an ordinary evening; Annie and the staff had planned something special—a talent show of sorts, where each resident could share a piece of themselves.

The room buzzed with quiet anticipation as chairs were arranged in a loose semicircle around a small makeshift stage. A microphone stood at the center, though Annie had reassured everyone that they didn't have to use it if they didn't want to.

Sarah was the first to step forward, her ever-cheerful demeanor lighting up the room. She clutched a children's book in her hands, the same one she had read earlier that morning. Her voice rang clear and steady as she read aloud, her words carrying a warmth that wrapped around the audience like a cozy blanket.

When she finished, the room erupted into applause. Sarah beamed, giving a small curtsy before taking her seat.

"You've still got it," Annie said with a wink.

Next came John, who approached the stage with his crossword puzzle in hand. He cleared his throat and adjusted his glasses, his voice steady but deliberate as he shared a few of his favorite clues.

"'Three-letter word for a young goat?'" he asked, his gaze scanning the room.

"Kid!" several residents called out in unison.

John nodded, a smile breaking through his usual serious expression. "Exactly. That's what this place feels like sometimes—a room full of kids."

The audience laughed, the mood light and playful. John returned to his seat, his shoulders a little straighter.

Linda followed, her painting tucked under her arm. She held it up for everyone to see— a vibrant depiction of the bird she swore she had seen that morning.

"It might not be real to you," Linda said, her voice soft but steady, "but it's real to me. And that's what matters."

The room fell silent for a moment, the weight of her words settling over everyone. Then the applause came, warm and genuine. Linda smiled, a flicker of her old artistic confidence returning.

Edward's turn came next. He walked to the front of the room, holding a tray of freshly baked cookies. He didn't say much—he didn't need to. Instead, he handed a cookie to each person in the audience, his precise movements speaking volumes about his care and dedication.

"These are perfect," Margaret said, biting into hers.

"Of course they are," Edward replied, his tone gruff but proud.

Margaret stood next, holding a book she had taken from the library. She read a passage aloud, her voice calm and measured. The words spoke of resilience and hope, themes that resonated deeply with everyone in the room.

When she finished, she closed the book gently and said, "We're all still here, aren't we? And that's something."

Her words drew murmurs of agreement and another round of applause.

Henry approached the stage with his harmonica in hand. He hesitated for a moment, his eyes scanning the room. Then he raised the instrument to his lips and began to play. The melody was soulful and haunting, each note carrying the weight of a lifetime of memories.

As the music filled the room, the residents leaned in, their expressions softening. When Henry finished, the applause was thunderous. He nodded his thanks, his face unreadable but his eyes glistening.

Emily's turn followed. She stood slowly, her movements unsteady but determined. "I'm not much of a performer," she said, her voice trembling, "but I can still dance."

She swayed gently to an imagined rhythm, her movements jerky but filled with emotion. The room watched in silence, their faces alight with admiration. When Emily finished, Sarah stood and clapped the loudest.

"That was beautiful," Sarah said, her voice thick with emotion.

Robert came forward next, his notebook clutched tightly in his hands. He handed it to Annie, gesturing for her to read. She opened it carefully and read aloud:

"I shaped cookies today. They weren't perfect, but they were mine. Like my memories—fragile, imperfect, but still mine."

The room was silent for a long moment, the weight of Robert's words hanging in the air. Then, slowly, the applause began, growing louder with each second. Robert smiled faintly, his eyes shining.

Mildred was the last to step forward. She held her cane tightly, her steps measured as she approached the microphone.

"I don't have much to say," she began, her voice soft but steady. "But I walked here tonight. And that's something."

The simplicity of her statement brought tears to Annie's eyes. The audience clapped, their admiration evident. Mildred nodded, a small but triumphant smile gracing her lips.

As the evening wound down, Annie stepped onto the stage. "Tonight wasn't just about talent," she said, her voice filled with emotion. "It was about sharing pieces of ourselves—our stories, our joys, our struggles. And I want you all to know how proud I am to be part of this community."

The residents clapped, their faces glowing with a sense of unity. For a moment, the challenges of their conditions faded into the background, replaced by a collective sense of belonging.

Later, as the residents returned to their rooms, the echoes of the evening lingered in the air. Annie walked through the quiet halls, her heart full. She paused outside each door, thinking of the people inside—Sarah's cheerfulness, John's determination, Linda's creativity, Edward's precision, Margaret's wisdom, Henry's soulfulness, Emily's resilience, Robert's introspection, Mildred's quiet strength, Frank's humor, Patricia's grace, and Carlos's belief in second chances.

Each of them carried their own stories, their own struggles, their own light. Together, they formed a tapestry of human connection—a reminder that even in the face of memory loss, creativity, humor, and vulnerability could bind people together.

And as the night deepened, Willow Grove Nursing Home grew quiet, but it remained alive with the echoes of its residents' voices, their stories, their songs.

The Heart of "Remember Me"

"Remember Me" is more than a series of interwoven narratives; it is a reflection of the human spirit in the face of cognitive decline. The book uses the unique experiences of twelve residents at Willow Grove Nursing Home to delve into the varied and often misunderstood world of dementia. It is a journey through the many types of dementia and memory loss, illustrating how these conditions affect individuals differently while emphasizing their shared humanity and resilience. This final chapter is not just a reflection on the book's stories but an exploration of what the conditions mean, how they shape the characters, and how they reveal the richness of life even amidst struggle.

Understanding Dementia Through the Stories

1. Alzheimer's Disease: Sarah's Warmth and Joy

Alzheimer's disease is the most common type of dementia, characterized by progressive memory loss, confusion, and changes in personality. Sarah embodies the early-to-mid stages of this condition. She wakes up cheerful and ready to take on the day, often mistaking Annie for her daughter or recalling stories from her teaching days that may or may not have happened exactly as she remembers.

Sarah's story demonstrates the emotional truth of Alzheimer's. Even as her memory falters, her warmth and joy shine through. This reflects a key aspect of Alzheimer's: emotional memory often persists even when factual memory fades. Her interactions with others remind us that the person remains, even when the disease alters how they connect with the world.

2. Vascular Dementia: John's Determined Puzzle-Solving

Vascular dementia results from reduced blood flow to the brain, often after strokes, and can cause slowed thinking, memory lapses, and difficulties with planning or problem-solving. John's love of crosswords reflects his attempt to hold onto his cognitive abilities. His frustration at losing words or struggling with simple clues mirrors the emotional toll of vascular dementia.

Yet, John's determination to keep solving puzzles represents the resilience seen in many people with this condition. His story highlights how small successes—completing even part of a crossword—can provide a sense of accomplishment and identity.

3. Lewy Body Dementia: Linda's Artistic Reality

Linda's experience with Lewy body dementia (LBD) is marked by vivid hallucinations, fluctuating cognitive abilities, and moments of clarity. Her belief that she saw a parrot in the garden reflects the condition's hallmark symptoms, where hallucinations can be so convincing that they feel real.

Her artistic expression becomes a way to process these experiences, turning what might be isolating into something beautiful. LBD often blurs the line between reality and perception, but Linda's story shows how creativity can serve as a bridge, allowing her to communicate her unique view of the world.

4. Frontotemporal Dementia: Edward's Search for Order

Frontotemporal dementia (FTD) primarily affects behavior and personality. Edward's impulsivity and fixation on reorganizing the kitchen are typical symptoms of FTD, where decision-making and social norms are disrupted.

Edward's story illustrates how individuals with FTD often seek control in their environment to counteract internal chaos. His precision in baking, a skill from his past, becomes a way to reconnect with himself and others. Through Edward, we see the tension between his changing behavior and his enduring skills, reminding us that dementia is not the absence of ability but its transformation.

5. Mixed Dementia: Margaret's Balancing Act

Margaret lives with mixed dementia, a combination of Alzheimer's and vascular dementia. This dual condition manifests in her difficulty navigating spaces and her moments of mental fog. She frequently gets lost, both physically and in conversation, yet she retains a deep sense of calm and connection.

Her librarian past and love for books anchor her, providing her with moments of clarity and purpose. Margaret's story underscores the complexity of mixed dementia, where symptoms overlap, creating unique challenges but also unique strengths.

6. Parkinson's Disease Dementia: Henry's Musical Memory

Henry's journey highlights the motor symptoms and cognitive decline associated with Parkinson's disease dementia (PDD). His tremors and difficulty with movement contrast with his effortless ability to play the harmonica, a skill deeply ingrained in his muscle memory.

Music becomes Henry's way of connecting with himself and the community. His harmonica-playing reminds us that while dementia may affect certain areas of the brain, others—such as those tied to music and rhythm—can remain remarkably intact. His story is a testament to the power of music to transcend cognitive limitations.

7. Huntington's Disease Dementia: Emily's Defiant Dance

Emily's erratic movements and emotional swings reflect Huntington's disease dementia, a condition marked by motor dysfunction and mood changes. Her decision to dance, despite her body's unpredictability, symbolizes her refusal to let the disease define her.

Emily's story is one of courage and defiance. Through her, the book illustrates how individuals with Huntington's can find ways to express themselves, even when their bodies and emotions feel out of control. Her dance is more than movement—it is a declaration of her enduring spirit.

8. Creutzfeldt-Jakob Disease: Robert's Notebook of Memories

Creutzfeldt-Jakob disease (CJD) progresses rapidly, causing severe cognitive decline and memory loss. Robert's reliance on his notebook to record fragments of his thoughts reflects the urgency and fragility of his condition.

His story emphasizes the importance of preserving memory, not just for himself but for those around him. The notebook becomes a symbol of his identity—a way to say, "This is who I am, even as I change."

9. Normal Pressure Hydrocephalus: Mildred's Steady Progress

Mildred's cautious steps and determination to walk reflect the effects of normal pressure hydrocephalus (NPH), a condition affecting mobility, memory, and bladder control. Her journey through the garden path mirrors her internal journey toward independence and self-assurance.

Mildred's story highlights the value of small victories. Her determination to walk, despite her challenges, serves as a metaphor for perseverance in the face of physical and cognitive decline.

10. Wernicke-Korsakoff Syndrome: Frank's Invented Realities

Frank's tendency to confabulate—filling memory gaps with fabricated stories—illustrates Wernicke-Korsakoff syndrome, often caused by a severe vitamin B1 deficiency. His humorous, exaggerated tales serve as both a coping mechanism and a way to connect with others.

Through Frank, the book explores the intersection of memory and imagination. His stories may not be factual, but they are true to his essence, showing that creativity can thrive even when memory fails.

11. Posterior Cortical Atrophy: Patricia's Blurred Perception

Patricia's difficulty recognizing images and faces reflects posterior cortical atrophy (PCA), a rare form of dementia that affects visual processing. Her connection to her photo album, despite her inability to see it clearly, symbolizes her emotional attachment to her memories.

Her story shows that even as perception changes, the heart holds onto what matters most. Patricia reminds us that memory is not just visual—it is deeply emotional and relational.

12. HIV-Associated Neurocognitive Disorder: Carlos's Second Chances

Carlos's fragmented memory and moments of clarity reflect HIV-associated neurocognitive disorder (HAND). His belief in second chances becomes a central theme, illustrating his efforts to rebuild his life despite the challenges of his condition.

Carlos's story highlights the intersection of stigma, resilience, and hope. Through him, the book explores how even fractured lives can find meaning and connection.

A Collective Tapestry

The residents of Willow Grove Nursing Home are individuals, each with their own story, but together they form a tapestry of shared humanity. Their interactions—Sarah encouraging Emily to dance, Linda's paintings inspiring Margaret, or Henry's harmonica uniting the group—show how community can uplift and sustain individuals facing memory loss.

The book demonstrates that while dementia affects cognition, it does not erase identity. Each character retains their essence, whether it is Sarah's warmth, Edward's precision, or Patricia's grace. These traits shine through their challenges, reminding readers that dementia does not define a person—it is merely one part of their story.

The Universal Themes

At its core, "Remember Me" is about connection, resilience, and the enduring power of the human spirit. It challenges stereotypes about dementia, showing that even in decline, there is room for growth, joy, and meaning. It asks readers to look beyond the condition and see the person—to honor their past while engaging with who they are in the present.

This book is a call to empathy and action, urging society to create environments where individuals with dementia can thrive. It is a reminder that every life, no matter how altered by illness, holds value and deserves to be remembered.

Made in the USA
Monee, IL
08 December 2024